Great HEALTH is WEALTH

STRATEGIES TO HEALTHY LIVING

YVONNE HOLALI HOTOR

Yvonne Holali Hotor

Table of contents

INTRODUCTION

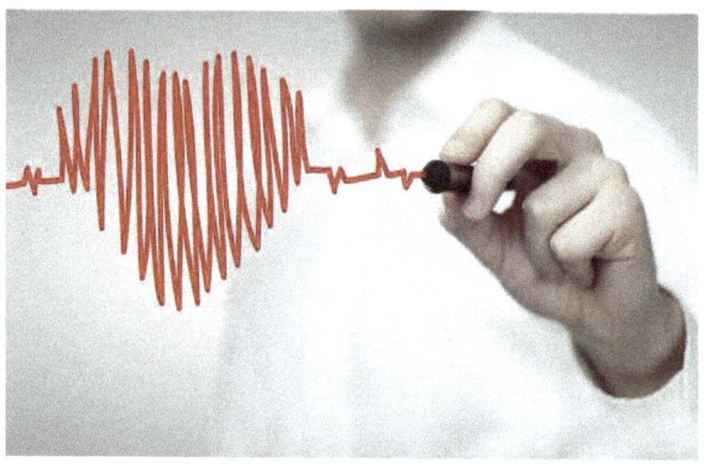

Lifestyle represents the set of actions and behaviors that you choose to put into practice in everyday life. It is natural that if we adopt healthy habits and therefore a healthy lifestyle, our body can benefit from it.

Why Having A Healthy Lifestyle Is Important

Having a healthy lifestyle is important not only to prevent possible diseases, but also to better enjoy the present and therefore your daily life. In fact, psycho-physical well-being is strongly correlated with lifestyle, what you choose to eat, how much you move and how you sleep. Although this close relationship between well-being and lifestyle is easily conceivable, in recent decades a new branch of science has been born, epigenetics, which deals with studying how the lifestyle and the environment in which one lives affect, directly with the expression of one's genes.

Certainly the genes that make up each person's DNA do not change over the course of life, but the way these genes manifest themselves can change instead. To better understand this phenomenon, it may be useful to consider the study done on two homozygous twins, that is, they have the same DNA. The two subjects involved, despite having precisely the same DNA and therefore, an equal genetic predisposition to develop some diseases, may then have very different problems throughout their lives.

This, as epigenetics explains, is due to the fact that individual behaviors and the environment in which one lives can make a difference in the activation or silencing of the genes that make up DNA. From this example we can therefore deduce that everyone can be partly responsible for their own well-being, choosing a healthy lifestyle and if possible an environment that helps them to live better.

How To Start Having A Healthy Lifestyle?

Learning the importance of adopting a healthy lifestyle is certainly important, but many times people, despite being aware of it, are held back from changing their habits. In this regard, to make change easier, it is important to always keep in mind that:

You don't change your lifestyle in a day or even in a month. It is right for everyone to take their time, also because rapid upheavals are often the least lasting ones.

Choosing a healthier lifestyle does not mean not being able to do something anymore, but preferring one habit to another. It is not an imposition, but a choice that is made for one's own well-being.

Many times the mind creates false beliefs and so we convince ourselves that we cannot change anything in our daily life. Only by trying can one understand that it is possible.

What Are The Correct Habits Of A Healthy Lifestyle?

A healthy lifestyle is made up of many simple actions, which repeated every day then become many healthy habits. These habits cover four major areas, which become the 3 pillars on which a healthy lifestyle is based:

- Nutrition
- Physical activity
- Rest

Nutrition

As for nutrition, it would be appropriate to return to making vegetables the protagonist of our meals, accompanying them with whole grains and a healthy source of protein, such as fish, eggs or legumes. On the contrary, packaged products should be limited, too often rich in preservatives, sweeteners and poor quality fats. Another good habit is to always check the glycemic load of your meals, limiting refined cereals and their flours, sugar and all its substitutes.

Physical Activity

Proper nutrition should always be accompanied by regular physical activity. This does not imply that you necessarily have to play a sport, but the important thing is to keep your body fit, toned and flexible. Therefore, no special equipment is needed, just a little commitment and perseverance.

Rest

However, a healthy lifestyle cannot be separated from rest, even if this aspect is too often neglected. Instead, it is during sleep that the body regenerates, recovers and strengthens itself. For this reason, it is important to choose evening activities that help you sleep better. After dinner, you should therefore switch off from your daily activities and instead listen to a relaxing meditation or read a good book.

In addition to thinking about the quality of sleep, it would also be useful to dedicate a few hours a week to activities that help you switch off, both physically and mentally. In this regard, a return to nature can certainly be regenerating. Even simple walks in the woods or by the sea can be a real cure-all at any time of the year.

These general tips can then be modified and above all customized according to the different needs that each individual may have based on age, gender and the goals they set for themselves. Instead, what should always be kept in mind is that each person, with their own habits and lifestyle can improve their well-being, to live better and in health. Let's learn more about creating a healthier happier life!

Yvonne Holali Hotor

Chapter 1

A HEALTHY MORNING ROUTINE TO SET YOUR DAYS

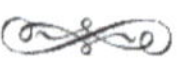

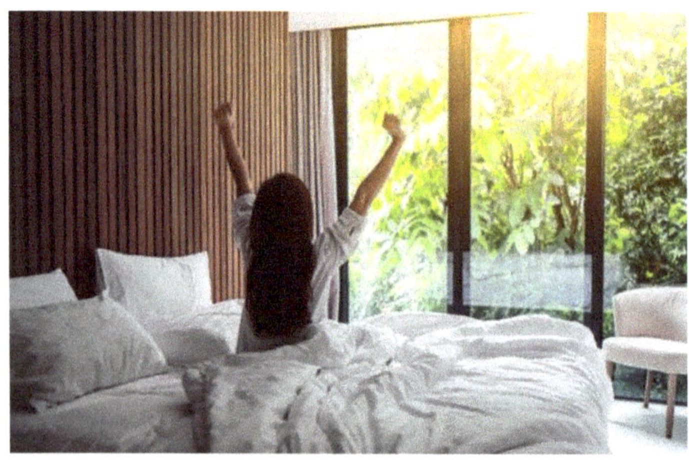

We always hear that a good breakfast is essential to start the day well, yet it can be done even better, it can raise the quality level of our entire morning routine, something not so simple and immediate but that, if you can to do, it can literally change our lives!

Culturally, we are inclined to pay more attention to the after-dinner, evening and nightlife (at least on weekends), but the real secret of our physical and inner well-being is instead to be found in the morning hours, from when we get out of bed. the first things to do.

So here are 5 rules to follow to try to get to organize a daily morning routine that can really make us make the leap in quality.

5 Basic Rules For A Perfect Morning Routine

As soon as you wake up, on an empty stomach, drink a glass of warm water with lemon; this purifies the intestine and prepares it to better assimilate the foods of the day, which will give you much more physical and mental energy.

After the glass of water and lemon, it is better to wait about 30 minutes before having breakfast, in order to give the drink time to act. This half hour can be used to do some physical activity, in order to awaken the body after hours of sleep. Doing physical activity immediately in the morning increases the strength to face the day and relaxes the brain and oxygenates it.

Turn on your pc and / or smartphone only after breakfast. Waking up and checking emails and messages immediately puts "others" at the center of our attention, thus increasing our state of stress and making us lose energy and attention for ourselves.

Have a real, healthy and hearty breakfast. Those who eat breakfast are less likely to be obese, have more stable blood sugar levels, and tend to be less hungry during the day. A healthy breakfast gives you energy, improves short-term memory, and helps you focus more intensely and for longer periods.

Set yourself at least one clear goal to achieve during the day. Having concrete goals enhances performance and also on an inner level you live better.

These are 5 activities to pay attention to and dedicate the right time every morning as soon as we get up. Being able to maintain this sequence over time will open the door to a better, healthier life, richer in energy and ideas and much less stressed.

Chapter 2

A POSITIVE MINDSET FOR OVERALL WELLNESS

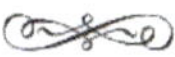

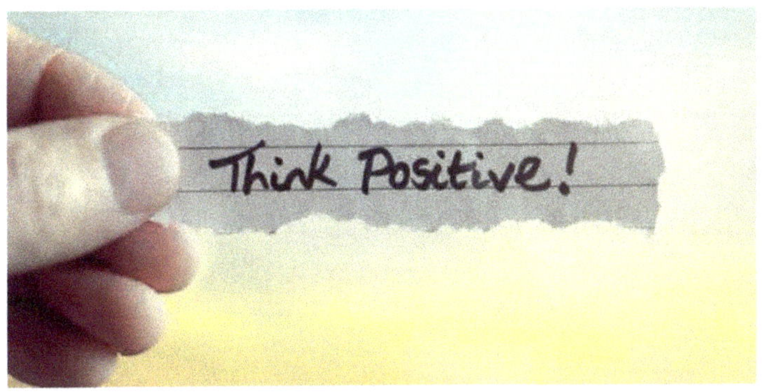

In the United States, the creation of the "Personal Development" interesting therapeutic proposal aimed at helping people to develop their potential; is a wonderful example to help understand the need to feel fullfilled. This need necessarily presupposes the identification of a series of objectives, such as having ideals, defining and planning goals, which must, however, be modulated while respecting one's limits and one's health.

Feeling fulfilled is a fundamental condition for the well-being of the individual as it is characterized by continuity over time and, therefore, by a sort of stability, the result of feeling in harmony with one's choices and with the consequences they bring.

In summary, this indicates the transition from what most European cultures call "positive thinking" towards what some other cultures call "Psychology of Wellness"; along this line, the optimistic vision of life is a mental strategy that facilitates the path towards the condition of emotional well-being as optimistic people consider situations with serenity and face moments of difficulty with a fighting spirit, patience and hope.

An optimistic attitude, in fact, can influence the choices of the individual and determine their success, as one does not give up in the face of difficulties thanks to greater mental strength than a pessimistic attitude.

Self-esteem is essential and, of vital importance, to our mental health.

"And do not be conformed to this world, but be transformed by the renewing of your mind, that you may prove what is that good and acceptable and perfect will of God."
- Romans 12:2 NKJV

Loving yourself must not be confused with selfishness or self-centeredness.

History, in fact, shows us that having self-love and being happy and satisfied with oneself are attitudes that, for a long time, have been underestimated and even judged negatively: "good and supportive people counsel each other out for the benefit of the other; you have to fight all forms of self-enhancement. At one time, there was a school of thought that self-care is sinful and led to impoverishing some internally because they distract us from the true path of internal development.

Today, however, enhancing one's self-esteem is one of the most important behaviors for achieving not only good satisfaction, but also a better quality in interpersonal relationships. "Self-esteem from within" is not a psychological state that arises spontaneously: it needs to be treated at all times, similar to the care of a mother for her own small child. In fact, the number of people who decide to commit themselves more to increasing their self-esteem is growing; self-esteem is, at this moment, a password that also in Italy represents the key to access happiness and well-being (as is further demonstrated by advertisements or course offers aimed at improving the individual).

Positively evaluating oneself allows the individual to be faithful to their principles, thus being able to feel strong and resistant, managing to assert their beliefs: this is the way to a full experience of personal fulfillment and, therefore, the way to happiness.

An optimistic attitude is relevant in this direction, leading to look at life in a totally positive way and to consider situations with serenity; optimism is a very important psychic strategy because it facilitates the path towards a state of psycho-physical well-being. In the field of psychology, various scientific researches have tried to find and understand the way in which an optimistic attitude, and in turn also a pessimistic one, can influence health and

psychological conditions; the conclusion of these studies is surprising
even if it may seem obvious, because it reveals that optimists are more successful than pessimists.

Optimism is a psychological state that consists in having hope and trust in what is about to happen and, therefore, knowing how to deal with events in a relaxed way, having a good mood, knowing how to laugh and look to the future lightly. One of the most important points of this attitude is that it inexorably pushes us to move forward; in fact, if we have a positive mood behind us, we are pushed to continue with courage, because we know with certainty that we will achieve success. All this makes us convinced and confident in our abilities by removing the fear of failure, fear, passivity and negative thoughts. The optimist considers failures to be transient, circumscribed and impersonal; so why not try to learn from failures, evaluating the mistakes made and above all the energy used considering that failure is an opportunity to learn, to grow and enrich one's experience, a challenge to carry out subsequent tasks in a better way.

Chapter 3

CHANGING HABITS

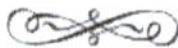

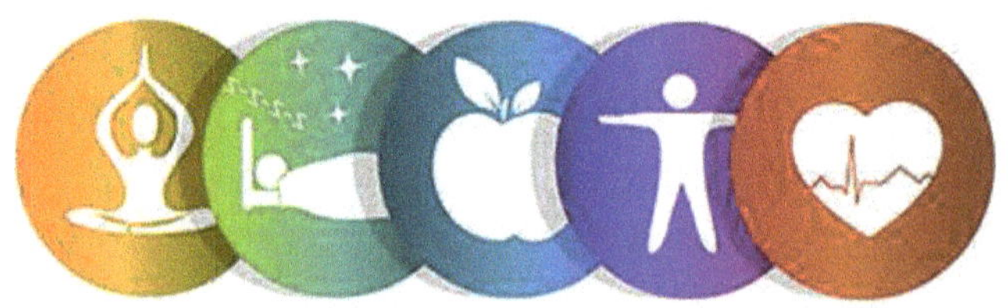

Each of us has different habits, which we automatically manifest during the day without awareness.

Many of the habits are harmful to health, such as: poor sleep, poor eating, drinking alcohol, smoking, sedentary lifestyle etc. Others constitute real obstacles to achieving goals, such as: being constantly distracted, procrastinating, justifying oneself, poor concentration, being disordered, wasting too much time in front of the TV or being on social media, etc.

The question we ask ourself is: But why is it so difficult to change a habit?

There are basically two reasons. The first reason is that habits have the power to change the structure of our brain. In fact, every time we behave in the same way, implementing a repetitive action, an automatic behavioral pattern is generated and strengthened in our brain. As long as our habits are healthy and useful, the automatic behavioral pattern that the brain puts in place can only help us harness our potential and change our lives. But, when habits are harmful, they can trap us in dysfunctional behavior patterns, which prevent us from improving by lowering our level of motivation and performance.

The second reason why it is difficult to change a habit is because our habits have created our zone of familiarity, that is, that safe place in which we feel protected, and in which we take refuge every time, that life places us in front of. a demanding challenge. Unfortunately for us, the familiar zone is a place where there is no possibility of growth, because we don't have new stimuli, and we don't go looking for it. All harmful habits keep us in this no-change zone.

To maintain enthusiasm and momentum high and to successfully achieve our goals, it is advisable for us to be able to change some habits. It is certainly not a change that we can make instantly, but if we clothe ourselves with willpower and perseverance, we will see the results.

Here Are Some Useful Tips For Changing Harmful Habits.

Become aware of your habits. A good idea is to write down your habits on a piece of paper, dividing them into good and bad. After that, try to identify the one that hinders your goal the most and replace it with a new, more useful habit. For example, if your goal is to lose weight, you might consider introducing a little more movement a day, for example with a walk, or avoid taking the elevator.

Build a morning ritual to develop positivity. Most people check their cell phones as soon as they wake up in the morning, and their minds are instantly bombarded with emails, notifications and news.

Then, they turn on the TV to watch the news full of bad news, and run out without having breakfast, perhaps just grabbing a coffee. This is a low-quality routine that doesn't make us start the day on the right foot. Recent studies in the field of behavioral psychology, however, have shown that a healthy morning routine allows you to start the day in a great way. Some of the benefits are: it clears the mind, improves the mood, improves energy and self-discipline, increases motivation and serenity. Some healthy morning habits you may start taking are:

Wake up 10 minutes earlier than usual and enjoy the silence by focusing on your breath and meditating on the word of God and prayer.

Wake up 30 minutes earlier than usual and do light gymnastics for 10 to 15 minutes
Waking up an hour earlier than usual and reading a good book for 20 minutes, or writing some creative ideas or writing down the most important goal of the day

Then, drink water, have a nutritious breakfast.

Choose the morning ritual that can have the most positive impact on you.

Change the triggers. Every habit action is activated by a trigger (trigger). For example, if you have the habit of smoking a cigarette immediately after coffee, coffee is the trigger that triggers your harmful behavior. Therefore, to reduce the likelihood of falling into automatic behavior, you will need to eliminate the triggers from the environment. If, in fact, we live in an environment in which the triggers to automatic behaviors no longer exist, the probability of adopting new habits increases. Therefore, if your goal is to quit smoking, and you are used to smoking after coffee, you can eliminate coffee, knowing that the urge to smoke a cigarette will be lower.

Train character and will. The impulses that lead us to perpetuate a habit are strong, so if we are not in control of ourselves, it is very easy to give in continuously to temptations. Therefore, if you really want to change a habit, at a certain point you will have to stand in front of the mirror, and ask yourself: "Who's in charge here?", Or "Who do I want to be in charge?"

Proceed gradually. The best way to fail is to believe that we can change everything in our life overnight. For example, if your goal is to be fit, you don't need to throw everything in the bin, but it is important that you introduce a small and simple new eating habit.

It must be something that you are convinced you can do and that should not be a burden to you. You will see that the satisfaction you will receive from making a small and simple change in your lifestyle will be enough to give you confidence and encourage you to make other changes.

Chapter 4

EMBRACING YOUR HEALTHIEST LIFE

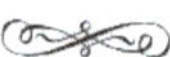

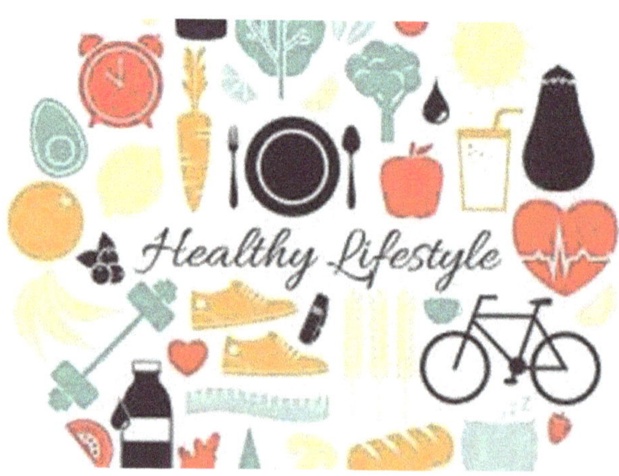

f like those readers, you too have a hard time finding direction in your life, start by giving yourself a goal, any goal, something you would like to accomplish, a good habit that you would like to form.

It does not matter. The first thing that comes to mind is fine, but dedicate yourself, with both your body and soul.

By doing so, you will give the first push to the "snowflake," triggering a virtuous circle.

Once you discover that you can achieve what you want, because you have decided, you will begin to enjoy it.

You will also want to better explore what your real desires are, what you want to be and become in life.

So let's give it this first push to the snowflake!

Below I have listed 100 good daily habits for you to start your new life in a positive way.

Don't worry, you don't have to establish them all or do all at once.

Remember: choose a first goal, any one, the one that will have inspired you the most at the end of this chapter and focus 100% on adopting this new behavior in your life.

As you adopt new healthy and healthy habits, as you reach your first goals, one after the other, you will begin to connect the dots and the direction in which you want to go in your life will become increasingly clear to you.

Are you ready?

So let's take this first step towards your new life. 100 good habits to change your life

Read this list head on and write down the habits that will motivate you the most, the ones that will make you feel a gasp inside, that will make you think "man, this thing I really want to do!."

Let's go!

Good Habits For Your Body

- Get up and move for at least 1 minute every hour (especially, if you are studying or doing sedentary work).
- Bring your heart rate between 50% and 70% of your maximum heart rate for 30 minutes a day.
- Spend 5 minutes doing exercises every morning to improve your flexibility.
- Leave your car in the parking lot farthest from the entrance to your office or shop.
- Take 10,000 steps a day.
- Take the stairs instead of the elevator.
- Eat an extra serving of fruit and vegetables a day with a morning smoothie.
- Drink the famous 8 glasses of water a day!
- Replace one of your daily coffees with a cup of green tea.
- Replace food crap with a healthier choice.
- Good practices for your mind

Good Habits For The Mind

- Read at least 2 pages of a personal growth manual every morning (hey, no one is forbidding you to read good fiction in addition, inspirational books with authentic word of God. I love it: but these two pages have a different function ...).
- Take 5 minutes each morning to imagine how the person you intend to become would live their day.
- Visualize the path to your most ambitious goals every day.
- Practice positive thinking daily
- Train your brain every day by solving sudokus, crossword puzzles and other mind games.
- Exercise your memory with the dictionary technique.
- Learn a new word of a foreign language every day.
- Listen to podcasts and audiobooks.
- In moments of transition (when you are on the road, while walking, while exercising, etc.) instead of using your smartphone absently, try to think deeply to find the solution to your problem or challenge.
- Use the trouble tree every night to get rid of your worries.

Good Habits For Your Spirit

- Meditate for at least 10 minutes a day.
- Write down 3 things that happened during the day every night that you feel grateful for.
- Perform a random act of kindness every day.
- Devote at least one hour a week to volunteering.
- Keep an effective journal.
- Immerse yourself in nature at least once a week.
- Spend 30 minutes on an activity without any specific purpose, which however makes you feel really good.
- Take care of an animal.
- Practice 4-step breathing daily.
- Put your problems in perspective by visiting this site at least once a week.

Good Habits For Your Productivity

- Use your smartphone for less than 60 minutes a day.
- Every Sunday make a rough plan of the activities for the following week.
- Make a detailed plan of the next day's activities each evening.
- Apply the tomato technique.
- Complete the most important, urgent and difficult tasks always first.
- Never check social media accounts or email as soon as you wake up.
- Use the Navy Seal alarm clock.
- Apply the single tap rule.
- Use your smartphone in black and white mode.
- Practice batching: Do similar tasks all at the same time of the day or week.

Good Habits For Your Wallet

- Automatically save at least 10% of your salary.
- Make a spending budget every month (and stick to it).
- Always postpone impulse purchases by 7 days.
- Delegate or ignore any activity that costs less than your ambitious hourly rate.
- Invest 15% of your salary every month in your personal training.
- Record all your income and all your expenses.
- Keep a journal of your financial decisions.
- Pay cash whenever possible.
- Work at least 30 minutes a day on a project that can generate an alternative source of income.
- Read an article on money management every week.

Good Deeds For Your Relationships

- Practice radical honesty on a daily basis: in other words, never lie, even for good.
- Keep the negative things to yourself and share the positive ones.
- Make at least a small "deposit" into the trust's current account every day.
- Smile when you meet other people's eyes.
- Make a commitment to remember the name of every new person you know
- Make anyone you meet feel appreciated and learn to use more phrases like: "Excuse me for the trouble", "You would like to be so kind ...", etc.
- Create a spark of romance in your love affair every day.
- Arrange at least one weekly appointment with your partner.
- You regularly hear from your friends, especially distant ones.
- Always follow up after a meeting. Develop the habit of sending a short message of thanks after a business or business meeting (in reality it does not hurt to do so also for friendships).

Good Habits For Your Career

- Think every day of at least 1 thing that can increase revenues, decrease costs or make life easier for your boss; then discuss it with the right person and take responsibility for implementing it if necessary.

- Take stock of the situation every month on your career path, clearly define where you want to go and talk about it whenever you have the opportunity with those who make the decisions in your company. To get anything, you must first learn how to ask.

- Constantly network internally (with your colleagues, with your superiors, with colleagues from other offices) and externally (with contacts from other companies in your sector or another sector in which you would like to work).

- Regularly ask for feedback on your work and implement any necessary improvements.

- Do at least 15 minutes of personal and professional training every single day.

- Read 1 article a day on the evolution of your professional sector.

- Always keep your CV up to date and if you don't have new experiences with which to update it every 12-18 months, ask yourself what's wrong with your career.
- Learn to negotiate: whether it's for a raise, annual bonus or benefit, always bargain.

Don't overdo the promises you make to your boss or customers, but then consistently exceed their expectations.

Practice your assertiveness every day.

Good Habits For Your Self-Esteem

- Face something that scares you every day (a little fear is enough: you don't need to jump out of a plane without a parachute).
- Apply the "as if" technique daily.
- Make your bed every morning. Starting the day with control over a small area of your life will help you face the rest of the daily challenges with the right attitude.
- Speak more slowly.
- Help someone who needs it, even a stranger. It will make you feel good and give you more self-confidence.
- Set yourself daily goals that push you to the edge of your skills (and stick to them).
- Keep the promises you make to yourself and others.
- Keep your shoulders straight
- Look after your appearance.
- Read Henry Ward Beecher's story at least once a month.

Good Personal Practices

- Always arrive 5 minutes early for appointments.
- Prioritize the quantity and quality of your sleep.
- Go to sleep earlier and wake up earlier. Because remember: an hour in the evening does not have the same quality as an hour in the morning.
- Get rid every day of an object that you do not usually use and that does not inspire joy in your life (this is an excellent habit to approach minimalism).
- Brush your teeth for at least 2 minutes a day, 3 times a day (and floss!).
- Every hour look at a point in the distance for at least 10 seconds (especially if you work all day in front of a screen).
- Wash your hands every time you go to the bathroom, touch raw meat, sneeze, or come home.
- Stop biting your nails.
- Learn to be tidier by "finding a place for anything and putting everything back in place" (after using it).
- Do not miss the opportunity to use the 3 magical expressions: "thank you", "please", "please".

Good Habits For Your Personal Growth

- Stop Whining: Whenever you are about to complain about something, force yourself to think about the solution to that same problem instead.
- Do not criticize and do not judge (neither yourself nor others).
- Stop watching the news
- Sign up for a course to learn a new skill.
- Attend a cultural event organized in your city at least once a month.
- Complete something imperfect every day: better an imperfect draft, than a perfect blank sheet.
- Identify your core personal values and live each day in line with these values.
- Create your own vision board and find inspiration and enthusiasm by staring at it every morning.
- Do your best every day with what you have available at that moment in terms of time, energy and other resources.
- Avoid zero days.

Chapter 5

YOUR MENTAL HEALTH MATTERS

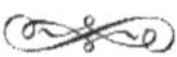

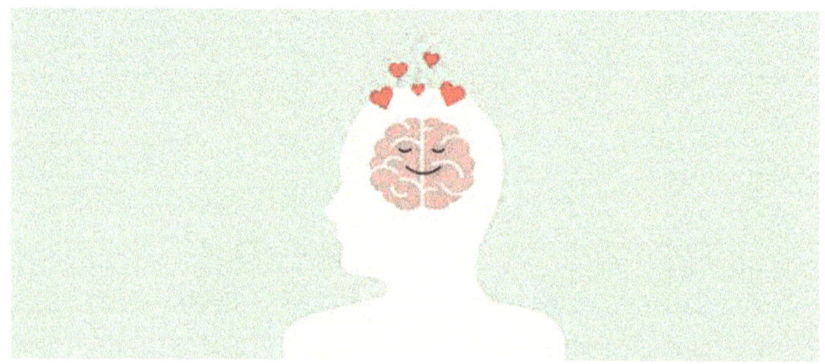

Taking care of your mental health is as important as taking care of your physical health. Some daily habits can contribute to the maintenance or improvement of one's psychological well-being.

It's about adopting a positive attitude and engaging in activities that promote mental health. Strengthening our personal emotional stamina i.e. our strengths and what makes us feel good, prepares us to better face the critical periods that may arise during our own life experiences

The following items are not a "magic recipe" for feeling good, but are simply some precautions that can contribute to mental well-being.

Recognize Your Strengths And Respect Your Limits

In modern society, performance and excellence have a high value. Yet the human being is not perfect and can be fragile. It is normal not to always be efficient, happy or brilliant.

It is important to take the time to get to know yourself better (for example through some reading, dialogue with family members or with a professional). This allows you to identify your abilities and accept your limitations.

Working through life events on an emotional level is a normal, necessary process and not necessarily a symptom of a disease. This process can also take some time. This is why it is important to be indulgent with yourself. When you feel the need, you can ask for support from your entourage or from specialists.

Take Care Of Yourself And Your Body

Taking care of yourself is a very personal thing. The means available are many and each must refer to those that suit him or her best. Physical activity is a useful tool to combat tensions, whether it be practicing a sport or taking a walk to take a breath of fresh air. The important thing is to do some movement, leave the house and change the air.

The activity phases can be followed by rest phases. The moments of rest allow you to "switch off" and therefore to calmly reflect and appreciate the events of the day. Although sleep is important, going out alone or in company and in a different atmosphere can promote relaxation. A fulfilling sex life if married or a well-lived spirituality can also be beneficial for mental health.

Cultivate Creativity And Individual Skills

The imagination and skills present in each are often just waiting to be expressed or developed. It is never too late to try your hand at a new activity and discover a new pastime or resume training.

Creative activities allow you to express positive or negative emotions without using the word. This allows you to dissolve tensions or worries.

Learning something new and developing your skills stimulates the mind, strengthens self-esteem and breaks the daily routine. This can be useful, for example, also on a professional level.

Countries, states, municipalities and cities often offer a rich program of cultural, artistic, sporting activities or training offers for adults. Some are free. Several organizations can offer support to people with modest income. Do not hesitate to inquire in your region.

Establish And Cultivate Social Relationships

The human being is a social being who is also realized through relationships with others. There are people who need social relationships more than others. It is important and useful to cultivate relationships with your entourage, whether it is family, friends, neighbors, or other members of society.

In some cases you can rely on friends to share joys and sorrows. It is important to find the courage to take a step towards others and open up to establish relationships, even if it is not always easy.

Speaking and listening allows you to put your ideas in order, helps to ease tensions and provides some relief. Sometimes talking about your concerns with someone else provides a new point of view and helps you find solutions.

There are also so-called self-help groups, which offer various forms of support. During peer interactions i.e. people with common view point or working situations; you can talk about your concerns and feelings. Generally this exchange gives the feeling of being understood without being judged.

You can also talk about your problems with different professionals whose job is to listen and give support in the search for suitable solutions. Asking for help is not a sign of weakness, on the contrary.

Chapter 6

POSITIVE VIVES FOR BETTER HEALTH

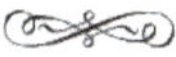

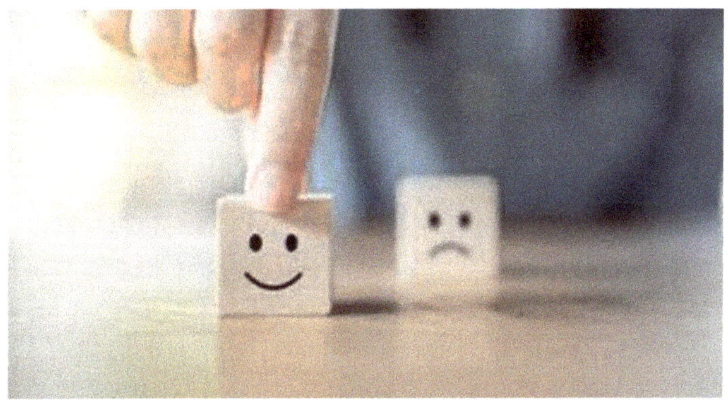

Do you want to have 5 to 10 years of extra life? Earn more? Succeed and realize your potential? Complete your projects? Simply the trick or secret to this life of success by some measures is called Positivity.

Norman Vincent Peale wrote: "Every event that concerns us is not as important as the attitude we have towards it, because that determines our success or our failure. How you think about a fact can defeat you even before you do anything about it. You are overwhelmed by events because you think you are. "

So the reasoning "when I will be well and when I earn more I will be more positive towards life" does not work. Instead it is exactly the opposite. Make an effort to have a positive attitude, to believe in it and to see yourself already winning in what you want. As a result, you will be in better health and earn more. It is proven. Let's see why:

The attitude of those who think positive is more suitable for dealing with life's challenges, rather than worrying. This can lead to fewer cases of disease. Studies have revealed that positivity makes it less prone to cardiovascular, gastrointestinal and even respiratory system disorders. Since the body is much more relaxed, the blood flow within the different systems is adequate and free.

Positive thinkers have more energy for worthwhile activities, good works and community outreach activities. They are able to cope with stress, and have constructive activities and eventually mental health improves. Positive thinking simply makes you more resilient and flexible in dealing with life's difficulties and problems. Adversity in life will come, it is sometimes unavoidable; however, those with a positive attitude face adversity differently. There is always something to be gained in experience from winning or losing. The word failure does not exist in the positive vocabulary. Sometimes, negative results make even determination stronger. The reason is that the positive brain feels compelled to seek other solutions creatively. It has no time to get depressed. The question is "What can I do?" Physically and psychologically, a person is much healthier when they have a more positive outlook on life.

Michael Steger and Todd Kashdan conducted a study in 2007. Participants kept records of their daily activities, along with their corresponding emotions each day for 21 days. The findings have simply shown that those who are often curious also gain more satisfaction with their lives and have a greater tendency to simply do activities that make them feel happy. Curiosity is simply defined as the state where you want to know more about something or someone. The reward after satisfying the curiosity provides the person with such a sense of accomplishment and a feeling of satisfaction.

Do you want to earn more? Your positive attitude can do this for you too. The researchers published a study on the link between cynicism and economic success in the Journal of Personality and Social Psychology. They evaluated data from around the world and found that high levels of cynicism are associated with lower income. The study reports that after nine years the cynical participants earned three hundred dollars a month less than their more positive counterparts.

British University of Warwick researchers Andrew J. Oswald, Eugenio Proto and Daniel Sgroi have conducted research on the effects of a positive mind in the workplace. In three different experiments, people selected at random and stimulated to positivity had about 12% more productivity.

Abraham Lincoln wrote: "Most people are as happy as they make up their minds to be." It's a choice. In other words, how can you change the narrative and be practical in creating good health because is wealth.

So here are 10 practical steps for positivity

1) Surround Yourself With Positive People

Much depends on who you hang out with. Possibly avoid or reduce contact with those who do not believe in you and only provide you with less constructive criticism, essentially trying to sabotage you. Negativity is as contagious as positivity. Those who do not believe in themselves want to console themselves with a large company of depressed people. People's negativity is toxic. They are not bad, but they have decided to be unhappy and to bask in this feeling. Others are envious of those who want to succeed and those who succeed. Don't go into that chicken coop if you want to fly high like eagles. Rather, it continues for a while on its own. Then you will find other eagles. Good flight.

2) Commitment

When we are given a task, no matter how big or small, we must take responsibility with total commitment. When we show commitment and enthusiasm to work towards our goals while ignoring failures and obstacles, we are truly able to attract and win the trust of the people who participate and support us in achieving our goals.

3) Conviction

To start thinking positively, you need to believe in yourself. It doesn't matter what the circumstances are. The first thing to do is believe that you can easily handle the situation. A negative mind will find many excuses and reasons to let go. Our belief in achieving a positive result will actually help us to continue to take on new challenges. Self-confidence helps you to take those first fundamental steps necessary to achieve success with effort and patience. No to haste!

4) Trust

Our brain hates unanswered questions, so it will lead us to try to predict future outcomes. How do we face the uncertainty of an unknown future? We usually divide life into two dimensions: good and bad. Let's avoid the uncertainty in between. Yet that's where we live. We simply live between the past and the future. The past can sometimes be the realm of wounded minds, and the future is still uncertain. It is today that we can easily begin to transform from the caterpillar of the past to the butterfly of the future. Believe it now.

5) Visualization

Visualization is one of the most fantastic and effective positive thinking techniques for achieving positive results. We can easily use it to imagine our dreams and desires and the success we wish to achieve. The visualization technique comes from our inner selves which actually makes us see the outside world differently. Negative thinking can also be a result of our visualizations and can create negative results. To practice this technique you can easily take pictures of what you want and keep them in the places you have the most frequent in your home in your daily life. When you see positive images daily, they will automatically help your subconscious become more positive.

6) Keep Your Inner Dialogue Under Control

Words have great power. An almost magical power (it is no coincidence that ancient spells were made of words). The words you say to others to support them or (sadly) to discourage them. The words you think about yourself are important. Avoid thinking in terms of "now", "what if...", "who, me?", "I'm too old or too young", "I don't know", "I'm not worth it", "I'm a nobody." You are sabotaging yourself. Do not think in terms of "if", but "when", already assuming that you will succeed. Say to yourself victory phrases and believe them. You will feel better and you will find winning solutions. For instance, this is how your day starts by getting upset at the alarm clock or someone. What would be the result of an athlete who competes already convinced of losing? Be determined to win, no matter what with your inner self.

7) Security

When you are endowed with confidence, you will feel like you have an invisible power. When you feel it, no pessimism can enter your life because you know you can get what you want out of your life. Trust dispels fear, the cause of our doubts. Think about your tomorrow and live in the present. Things can go wrong and they won't always go as planned. However, never expect them to go wrong. Don't accept defeat from whatever bad things can happen. When it goes wrong, you understand why. The crucial thing is how you deal with negative feedback and start running again.

8) Set Specific Goals And Write Them Down

A goal must be "SMART" meaning: Specific, Measurable, Accessible, Realistic, and Timely with an expiration date. Changing your mind starts with a desire to do it. Desire alone won't help you become a positivity magnet. You also have to act. This basically means setting goals and taking steps to achieve your goals. The most effective way to achieve a larger goal is to break it down into smaller goals. This will allow you to proceed knowing that you are one step closer to achieving your greatest goal.

9) Think Big

Having realistic goals does not mean being satisfied with little. Fuel your self-esteem, nurture your creativity, and strive to achieve great goals by stepping out of your comfort zone. Challenge yourself to be the best of who you can be. Those who are satisfied do not enjoy, they resign themselves. And this is certainly not a positive attitude. Never envy anyone for any reason. It makes you feel inferior. Take an example, study the story of successful people, adapt it to yourself and never think that you are less than them (especially without knowing the sacrifices they went through to get there).

10) Avoid What Reminds You Of Failures And Boredom

A place or an object can remind you of the past. They can be harmful, especially when you are trying to forget a sad event in your life that you may have been through. Take them off. Boredom is also to be avoided. When you are bored and have nothing to do, your mind wanders and can lead to unhappy thoughts. It is vital to keep yourself busy and productive so that those negative thoughts don't enter your mind. Use the time to study, to grow, meditation, prayer, and to reach your super version. "Change your thoughts and you will change your world."

CONCLUSION

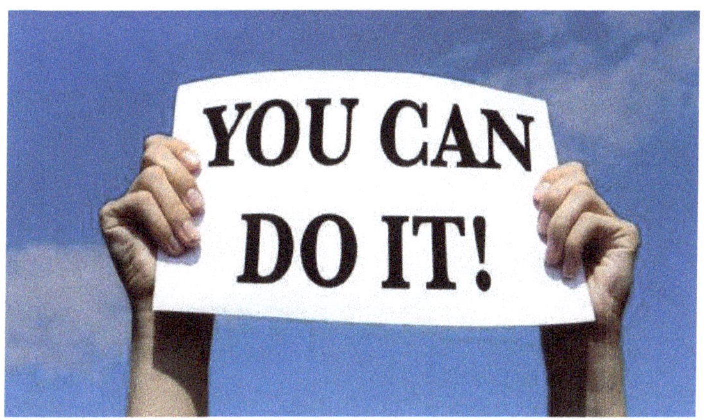

it seems really elementary and logical, but we often find ourselves embroiled in a negative life condition and we don't realize that our efforts to get out of it are zero. We haven't even thought of a solution, lifted a finger, nothing. In practice, we are not doing anything that can give us hope for some improvement.

It is therefore first and foremost essential to understand if we really want to make a real change in our daily life. Is there this desire? Are you ready to collect and use all your energy to make it happen?

The point is, you can never change your life if you don't start changing the way you conduct your days. If there is something you don't like, if you want a different future, you have to face the fact that something needs to be changed to start engaging a transformation.

You have to find your motivation, your energy, your gasoline. You have to be 100% firm and sure that's what you want. Not because you won't be able to go back, but because otherwise it would be an incredible waste of time.

If you are convinced that you want to become the master of your future, start your journey. Look inside and evaluate what are your resources, your strengths, your real desires. Also consider what fears are holding you back and the excuses you tell yourself for never really facing your inner obstacles. Finally, set your goal and define as much detail as possible.

Don't be held back by the fear of making mistakes. And don't get lost in the "ifs" and "buts" loops. After all, it is always time to change course!

Yvonne Holali Hetor